Scientifically Proven Ways

to Grow Muscle Fast

Richard Perkins

Table Of Contents

Tips on How to Promote Muscle Growth Fast

Muscle growth is not just about lifting weights and going to the gym everyday but there is a science behind it. You have to remember that the body has certain ways on dealing with stress. Every person also has different metabolism rates, and because of this, they may need different exercise programs.

When it comes to body building, you should be able to know about the different theories concerning it. By knowing about the theories, you will be able to apply it in your exercise regime and get the results you want at a much faster rate.

For building muscles, you have to remember that resting is very important if you lift weights at the gym. Never ever exercise the same muscle group everyday unless you are concentrating on fat loss. However, if you want to gain muscle, resting the muscles is a very important part of it.

For example, if you exercise your chest today, don't exercise it tomorrow. This means no bench presses tomorrow.

You have to consider the fact that whenever we lift weights, we injure our muscles. Therefore, the body will react by fixing it with bigger and much stronger muscles. And, in order to promote muscle repair, we need to get some sleep and let the muscle we injure rest for at least two days.

Diet is also an important factor when you want to gain muscle mass. Always remember that protein is very important when it comes to muscle growth. Protein helps in rebuilding muscles and promote muscle repair. So, how much protein you should eat? Basically, the rule of thumb is that for every pound you weigh, you need at least 1.5 grams of protein. This means that if you weigh 200 pounds, you need to take in 300 grams of protein a day. That is if you work out regularly.

There are supplements that you may want to try. Some are rich in amino acids that also promote protein production and muscle growth, while there is also whey protein that directly introduces the needed daily protein intake in your body.

 If you want to gain muscle, another key is proper execution of exercises and the right exercises.

The right exercises for muscle gain are usually free weight exercises. As much as possible, you should do free weight exercises and minimize the use of machines. Although machines do lower the risk of injury, you have to remember that free weight is much more effective in promoting muscle growth. Always remember that in order to promote muscle growth, you also need to strengthen the supporting muscles. For example, if you want to promote muscle growth on your biceps, you also need to strengthen the muscles that surround the biceps.

And, only free weight exercises can do this. Machine exercises virtually does not put any strain on the supporting muscles, which means that it will not promote the growth of your primary muscles as well as free weight exercises can.

Proper execution of the exercise is also very important. By doing the exercises slowly and in a controlled and smooth motion, you will promote maximum muscle contractions which means that it will promote muscle growth.

These are just some of the many body building muscle gain tips that you need to keep in mind. There are quite a lot of techniques that will be able to help you gain muscle. With these tips, you will be able to get the body you want in no time at all.

A Gaining Muscle Primer for Teenage Boys

High school, most of us have many happy memories about it. Many of our most memorable experiences come from this carefree moment in our lives. And as each student prepare for this time of their lives, they also discover the joy of meeting the opposite sex. Teenage boys for one will do most anything to create a good impression and one of them is having a well chiseled body. This is when most teenage boys would think about working out and lifting weights.

Remember your own teenage years? Do you continually compare muscle gain with some of your friends? It was that then and it is still that way now. In fact, it is more prevalent today as more teenage boys are becoming more conscious of their bodies. There is simply no denying it; gaining muscle is the in thing.

As a parent, it is wise to support this mentality, not only will your teenage son be able have a healthier body, they will also develop self confidence. The problem is, some boys would go take the easier route. They would take steroids or whatever to help facilitate the fastest way in gaining muscle; this will not help them at all, especially in the determination and motivation department. As a parent it is their duty to show them the proper way to grow muscles.

The best way to gain muscles would always be the tried and tested means, the proper diet and a rigorous and painstaking weight lifting workout regimen. A proper diet will be determined if your son is overweight or underweight. In the first scenario, your kid should lose weight first and eliminate body fat. Muscle building will follow suit after at least a significant weight loss is experienced.

This diet would mean eliminating fats and calories; just enough should remain for fueling muscle growth. In the latter, it is the opposite, a skinny kid should eat more but should have the proper intake so that body fat is not created, rigorous strength training should be done simultaneously to build up bulk, mostly of muscles.

It is not advisable to immediately push a teenage boy into a full intense workout as their body is still developing. They should be gradually introduced in the program to allow their body to adjust. Make sure also that they have sufficient rest as teenage boys are a bundle of energy. Redirecting this energy in a well planned workout program will allow them to maximize the use of their energy.

Most importantly though it is the attitude that should be set first before embarking on a gaining muscle journey. Teenage boys are easily distracted and they can easily forget that they are working on a goal. They must be determined to finish what they will be starting. With full commitment, they will be able to achieve success in gaining muscle in no time at all.

These are just some of the things one must consider when starting a program of gaining muscle. There are lots more, but most importantly, it is all about discipline. Having a healthy and great looking body works wonders to a person, especially to a teenage boy. There is nothing quite like the present to start on this fruitful journey. So there you go.

Alcohol Can Ruin Muscle Gain

You heard it right. Alcohol is one of the major reasons for wasting your most beloved physique and muscles that you have taken care of for years. Alcohol is considered as one of the most significant causes to lose your muscle's nice features. Despite of what health experts are trying to imply about the negative effects of alcohol, others are still on the verge of tiring themselves with it. Drinking alcohol will definitely ruin muscle gain.

Alcohol is considered as one of the most influential drinks ever invented. Not that it tastes funny but also this drink can now be considered as a drug because of its addictive effects which can affect your life including your family, friends and work. If you really want to maintain your six packs (abs not beer) and your mass, you have to be conscious about drinking alcohol because it can cause deterioration of your years of fruitful labor. What are the effects of alcohol in your body?

1. Increases estrogen and decreases testosterone levels.
If you wanted to increase your muscles, then you have to maintain or increase the levels of testosterone inside your body because it is that hormone that can gear to building your muscles. It will be a loss on your part, as men, if you allowed estrogen to overcome your testosterone levels because that can also cause secondary female characteristics.

2. Affects protein synthesis, big time!

You know that protein is one of the most important nutrients that your body needs in order to gain those additional mass. When you hinder protein synthesis because of too much alcoholism, you tend to hinder for protein to be distributed all throughout your body. Protein synthesis will be slowed down for about 20% the normal status.

3. Strips the body of minerals and vitamins.
Alcohol has a diuretic effect on the body which promotes increase excretion of minerals and vitamins inside the body. When too much alcohol is consumed, it tends to strip off some of the important elements that our body needs namely Vitamin A, B complex, C, calcium, phosphorus and zinc. These elements are drained in rapid manner which can cause comprise to our body's balance. In order to function properly, one must maintain the sufficient amount of minerals and vitamins inside the body that definitely involves supporting muscle growth.

4. Dehydration can and will occur.
Haven't you noticed that every time you drink alcohol, you tend to ask for cold water or soda just to get rid of your thirst? This is because, as what is already said, that alcohol is fast-acting diuretic that can increase your body's ability to dispose water. No doubt about it, every time you visit the John, the essential vitamins and minerals in your body are lost in your urine. If this continues to happen, the water in your body can't sustain the necessity because of the increase excretion and muscle demand. And muscles are composed of about 60-70% water!

4. Increases storage of fats

Drinkers are known to possess large bellies. That's because alcohol can trigger deposition of fats inside our bodies. Alcohol contains about 7 calories every gram which is the main reason why alcohol can make people fat in an unnatural way.

You have to take care of how you manage drinking most especially if you are maintaining an ideal body weight and size. A few drinks occasionally aren't bad as long as you can handle the effects. Otherwise your muscle gaining goals can be totally affected in a very negative way.

Boost Your Metabolism While Gaining Muscles

Your body has a rate that metabolizes food into energy to be stored in forms of fats and glucose. The more your body increases its percentage of utilizing energy, the more your muscle gains mass. In order gain firm muscles, your body will have to adapt to the stress cast upon your body and muscles.

These instructions are of the moderate type. Following the ways will let you boost your metabolism and at the same time gain the muscle mass that you desire.

1. Do a 10-minute warm up. You can do a brisk walk in order to get blood pumping. This kind of warm up exercise can increase the amount of circulating blood inside your body. Muscles should always be nourished by free-flowing blood in order to maintain a good bodybuilding state. Your muscles will also become more receptive to any kinds of resistance.

2. Be sure that you target larger muscle groups in order to boost the level of your metabolism and provide the needed resistance your body needs to build the muscles. You have to maintain consistency in order for you to capture results in just a couple of months.

3. Start on your hips, buttocks and thighs. Do some lunges to raise the amount of your metabolic rate. You should first hold on to something hard

to be able to attain balance. As you build the muscles that you need, you have can now stick to supporting the lower part of your body and holding dumbbells to raise the muscle resistance and metabolism.

4. Stand straight then use the dumbbell which has the heaviest proportion that you can lift comfortably over the head. Grasp it at the level of your shoulder with the palm of your hand facing forward then push it overhead in a straight manner until your arm have reached its full extension before it returns from the position where you started. Do this exercise in 10 repetitions, slowly so that you will not strain your arm after which, switch the dumbbell to the other arm. Do the repetitions at least three times from either hands. You have to be sure that your body and arms can tolerate the repetitions otherwise you are prone to muscle wasting as well as injury.

5. Alternate exercises. For the last one mentioned, you can do the dumbbells and after several repetitions, go down with the push-up. This is very efficient because of the evident use in military training. Push-ups, in general, provides resistance to weight that is needed to build muscles and at the same time increasing the rate of metabolism. If you are having difficulties with push-ups, you can start with simpler ones like knee push-ups.

6. For other upper-body exercises, you can use the dumbbells so that you can target the shoulders, upper muscles of the chest, forearms and muscles of your deltoid. Dumbbells have greater chances of increasing the rate of your metabolism faster that other equipments do.

7. Lastly, consider to alter certain areas in your lifestyle that is in conjunction with the exercise that you are habitually maximizing. If you consume more fats before, then try toning it down to limited amounts. Instead, consume something that has a higher content of protein, calories and nutrients.

It is also good that you consume vegetables, whole grain and citrus fruits. This will give you more advantage for your muscle gaining technique.

Eat Right to Gain Muscles Correctly

Without proper diet, you can't expect to gain the muscle that you want. It is not enough to know all weight gain exercises to be able to achieve your desired muscle mass. You have to also be particular about what goes in and out of your body. Diet will support your bodybuilding methods. Here are some ways to ensure that you acquire the correct diet in you weight gain activity.

Get at least two times your body weight

For example, if you weight 100lbs, you must eat a diet that will give you at least 100 up to 200 grams of protein so that you are assured to obtain muscle growth consistently. For those who are into full time bodybuilding, it is advised that you consume 2 to 3 times your bodyweight in regards to protein.

Protein varieties should be considered

You should a have protein varieties to consider. One of which is red meat which is rich in protein although there are also alternatives like fish. Cottage cheese, soy, nuts, beans and rice are all rich in protein. On the other hand, these products have different kinds of amino acids which is why varieties are much, much better.

Supplements are good

Other sources of protein can be taken from supplements wherein you don't have to buy meat just to attain the required protein in your everyday consumption. Soy proteins and whey are some of the common examples. You have to make sure that when you incorporate these in your meal, increased fluid intake must be assured or else it will strain the kidneys or liver and will contribute to a certain impact on the part of the organs. Increased fluid intake will be helpful in flushing out the negative effects of consuming high protein.

Balance

If you are doing a strenuous routine or anything aerobic, if you don't eat a diet that is high in protein it will cause your muscles to lose its strength and mass. There are numerous college and even high school athletes that are faced with muscle strength that are declining through the season of their game because they are unaware of this fact. Following this will not do any harm and instead becomes advantageous.

Carbs galore

Carbohydrates should always be included in your diet because it's responsible for the energy that you exert when you lift weights or any heavy object. You will not be pumped up without taking in carbs with your proteins. Carbohydrate is one essential element needed in the production of energy.

Words of advice:

• Drink loads of water to be able to replace the fluid that was lost in your body and to eliminate the waste product of protein metabolism. This will also prevent your high-protein diet from harming or damaging your organs and is actually helpful to make you lose weight.

• Calories must be minimized if you really want to gain the weight that you desire. It will be difficult on your part to exert a lot of efforts without gaining anything.

• Never consider taking steroids. It will only give you more negative than positive effects. You should consider gaining muscle the natural way so that measures will be healthier on the part of your body. Even health experts won't advice the use of steroids because of the numerous negative side effects that one can get.

Eating More to Gain Muscle

That doesn't sound right, does it? Most people go on strict diets when developing their body. A lot of us dream of having a healthy and great looking body. Some spend countless hours in the gym, and spend thousands of dollars on equipment just to gain muscles. Some people even have medicine cabinets lined up and filled to the brim with gain muscle medications and supplements. The fact is, a lot of these people find the process too tedious and too slow.

Going back to eating more for gaining muscle, this may sound incredulous to some as popular notion would have people cutting back on their food intake so that body fat will be diminished allowing muscles to be more pronounced. As there are more body fat covering the muscles, they are not able to fully expose all the cuts and lines that give the body muscle definition.

But we have to remember that as we cut off our calorie intake, you are not giving your muscles the proper nutrition it needs to help make them grow bigger. What you need to do is to increase your calorie intake if you want to gain weight, but this pertains to gaining weight because of muscle development, and not body fat. Ingest proteins and fats to provide your body all the calories it requires to gain muscle but be wary in ingesting too much calories because then the result would be the development of body fat.

This is where having a good workout routine comes in. As you do your regular workout, targeting the muscles which you want to develop, you will be able to burn all the calories you have ingested allowing it to go to your muscles to help them develop, and at the same time, avoid them into turning into body fat.

For faster muscle gain and growth, do workouts that include heavy weights. Be very patient and persistent. Some people tend to give up as frequent lifting of heavy weights can literally be a pain. If you are not accustomed to lifting weights, then it's highly likely that you will feel soreness in your muscles. This is natural; in fact, this is one way your body is telling you that your muscles are growing, think of it as growing pains.

Weight lifting will promote muscle gain and as you eat more, the increased caloric intake will supply the boost your body will need to promote the growth of muscle tissues. When building muscle tissues, you will also be gaining strength. If you diet too much and not have the proper food intake while weight lifting, you will just lose muscle instead of your goal of building them. Doing free weight exercises in addition to lifting heavy weights will help in gaining muscle faster. Your body will be able to quickly respond in its process of building muscle.

So how much is eating more and yet not gaining body fat? That all depends on you, your body structure will determine this. A nutritionist will be able to determine how much calorie intake you will need in gaining muscle.

With a steady food intake specially developed for you and a proper workout, you will soon be able to develop the body you have always wanted and also gain the self confidence and pride that will make you feel a whole lot better about yourself.

Exercises That Will Promote Muscle Gain

Have you ever wanted to have that body that you can be proud of? Do you want to confidently walk around the beach with your shirt off? If you answered yes to any of these questions, then what you want is to gain some muscles or to have a muscular or ripped body.

If you want to get a ripped body, then you definitely need to go to the gym and start lifting weights. However, you have to remember that lifting weights alone will not promote muscle growth. There are basically lots of things that you need to consider when you go to the gym and when you want to build muscles. First of all, not all exercise programs are designed for body building. Also, not all exercises are effective in promoting muscle growth.

If you really want to gain muscles, then here are some body building tips that you need to remember.

First of all, body building is basically a three day exercise regime. On the first day, you should try exercising the chest and the triceps. You should at least do four exercises for each muscle group. For the chest, you should do the bench press, inclined barbell press, lying dumbbell fly, and cable crossover. For the triceps, try the kickbacks, barbell triceps presses, close grip bench press, and V-Bar pull down.

For the second day, work your back and biceps. For the back, you can do the bent over barbell row, Romanian dead lift, dumbbell lying row, and cable seated row. For the biceps, you can do the alternate dumbbell curl, standing barbell curl, preacher curl, and cable curl.

For the third day, work on the legs and shoulders. For the legs, you should do the squats, leg press, leg extension, and seated calve raises. For the shoulders, do the barbell behind neck press, military press, Arnold press, and shoulder press.

For every exercise, you should do at least 3 sets with 10 repetitions for each set. You should also remember that in each day, you should exercise your abdominal muscles with sit ups, weighted knee raise, and hanging leg raise. For each exercise, you should do at least 2 sets with 30 repetitions each.

These are samples of the exercises that you should do. You can work out 3 times a week or if you have time, you can work out 6 times a week with Sunday as your rest day.

It's usually up to you on how you schedule your workout regime. However, you have to remember that you shouldn't forget to rest. And, you have to have adequate sleep in order to promote muscle growth. Another thing that you need to remember is not to do the same exercises for two consecutive days.

Also, every two weeks, you might want to change the whole program with whole new sets of different exercises for the same muscle group. You will see that there are quite a lot of exercises that you can do.

Remember these tips and you can be sure that you will be able to promote muscle growth or muscle gain. As you can see, it is quite easy for you to build muscles on your body. All it takes is dedication and proper execution of the exercises. In just a short time, you will see positive results with your body.

Exercises to Effectively Increase Bicep Muscle Mass

Have you ever wanted to have a great looking body that you can be proud to show off in the beach? First of all, muscle gain is different from weight loss. You have to remember that there are quite a lot of exercises out there that are designed to target different parts of the body. Some exercises are targeted for fat loss, while there are others that targets muscle gain.

If you want to gain muscles, then here are some exercises that you may want to know about which can help you gain muscle mass in just a short period of time.

For starters, the biceps are the most sought after muscle group that most people want to build up. Besides, you would definitely look great if you had big biceps, wouldn't you? So, here are some of the exercises that you may want to know about in order for you to gain muscles on your biceps.

The first exercise that you should do is the standing bar curls. With a barbell curl, you will be able to directly target in exercising the biceps. You will be injuring the biceps more, which means that it will allow you to build up your muscles in your biceps.

To do this exercise, you need to stand with your feet at about shoulder width apart. Hold the bar with an underhand grip. The starting position is where you are standing as instructed, and the arms should be straight with the biceps fully extended. Your upper body should be leaning slightly forward and with one explosive motion, curl your arms with the weight concentrating on your biceps.

Then, you have to remember that when you go back to the starting position, you need to extend your biceps slowly. Remember that lowering the weight actually is more effective than the actual curl. Lower the weight slowly and not just drop the weight all the way down.

If the straight bar is putting a lot of stress on your wrists, which for some people does, then you might want to try the EZ bar curls. This will put your wrists in a much comfortable position and will help you lift the weights much easier and in a much comfortable way but will not decrease the overall impact on your biceps.

Standing alternate dumbbell curls are also a great way to build muscles in your biceps. What you do is hold one dumbbell on each hand at your sides with the palms facing each other. Then, curl one dumbbell at a time and at the same time rotate your palm forward as you lift. After you fully contract the biceps, lower the dumbbell with the arm rotating back to its original starting position. Do this with your other arm. That's basically it. You don't need any machines or special benches to do these exercises.

For both exercises, you might want to do 10 repetitions with 3 sets.

The key here is to overload your biceps. After exercising your biceps, you have to let it rest for at least two days. You need to remember that when you lift weights, you are actually injuring your muscles in order for it to grow more muscles to support the weight you are constantly lifting. This means muscle gain.

Five Effective Ways to Gain Muscles

If you have spent all your life inside the gym just to find out that nothing's happening aside from muscle pains then you must be doing something really wrong. You have to assess yourself. Fact is, gaining muscle mass can't be done in just a day. You can't even see it coming even if weeks have already passed. Muscle gain is achieved only after months of rigid exercise and it requires lots and lots of devotion and determination in order for your body building program to work.

Either way, here are five of the most effective ways to help you boost up your knowledge and skills in totally achieving your muscle growth goal. You can choose to follow these tips or guidelines just in case.

Have a meaty diet

In order to increase the mass of your body, you have to increase protein intake. That would be simple, right? Meats should be categorized as red meat because they contain certain nutrients that are required for your muscles to grow. You don't need scientists to figure that one out. You just need to combine protein with the right kind of food like veggies or juice drinks which will help you to further acquire the buffer you need.

Use weights, the free ones

Here, you can use the usual dumbbells in order to add to the movements of your exercise. This equipment can also improve your ancillary muscles in order to have a wider range of motion. Free weights are also helpful in increasing the number of muscles that you want.

Safety first

Above all else, before and after you start your routine in the gym, you have to observe proper safety in order to avoid or prevent any injuries that may occur. When you're bodybuilding, be sure that you take it one step at a time. Don't combine heavy weight with intensive sessions of workouts because you make yourself more vulnerable to get injured. It's very common for bodybuilders to experience strains, torn and disc slips. You can avoid these things from happening just by being more aware of the different precautionary measures. You also might want to warm up so that your body's circulation will be more efficient once you start the real session.

Flirt with alternatives

If you think that you already have met your requirements for your body, you can do other maximums in order to assess yourself. This will give you the opportunity to check the status of your overall strength. However, when you do something more strenuous, you have to make sure that your muscles can handle the stress otherwise it will have a negative feedback on your muscles. Thus, in the duration of your bodybuilding time, you are still expected and recommended that you increase the weight.

Observe for improvements

In order to assess that you have achieved something, you have to determine how far you've come. You can check your present status from other people or muscle teams. This will teach you other terms on how to improve some areas of your strengths and weaknesses. In observing people, you will be able to see how far you've come in gaining muscle mass or how much more there is to do.

Comparison is always effective to improve someone's ideals and capabilities.

Gain Muscle and be a Fashion Icon

Gaining muscle mass is considered as one of the dreams of every male all over the world? Why? It adds up to their masculinity and makes girls want them and gain more confidence. Admit it, if you're still in high school and someone asks you about what you want your body to look like, you'll choose the jock that has a pea for a brain but a body of a ramp model rather than a geek hiding underneath glasses who's a walking encyclopedia. But really, gaining muscle isn't all for those who can't gain brain. It's just that, some would compensate gaining muscles rather than knowledge.

Much said. Would it be nicer if you have hunk-like muscles and a very intelligent personality? You're like a walking package. Women love muscles more than an intelligent mind, well, not entirely. But most of them do. On the other hand, gaining muscles is for those who are conscious about their body. With the trend of having nice abs and mass, it would be nice if people see gaining of additional mass as something healthy and not just to prove masculinity.

Let's face it. Because of the appearance conscious society that we live in today, some men result to drastic measures in order to maintain their supple physique even with the absence of exercise. If you are that type who uses artificial products like steroids, then it's time that you renew your ways because there is no way that you can get something out of nothing.

There is a natural way of having the muscles that you love to have. You just have to be more committed and disciplined in order to follow the ideal way. Here are some of the most important tips in order to shape yourself up.

1. Modify your diet.

It is not enough that you exert so much effort in bodybuilding. You also have to maintain the required dietary allowance that you need in order to be in top shape. Easting foods which are rich in fatty acids (omega-3) and fish are rich in protein and will help you grow. Some of the fish which are rich in omega-3 are lake trout, salmon, herring, mackerel, sardines and tuna.

Veggies or plant crops which are also rich in omega-3 such as walnuts, broccoli, cauliflower, cabbage, spinach, soybeans, tofu and kale can also be included in the diet. Foods rich in omega-3 provide our muscles sensitive to insulin which help to fuel glycogen storage and hinder entry of amino acid into muscles.

2. Intake of sodium.

To encourage the growth of your muscles, you should increase healthy sodium intake in order to increase the fluid of your muscles. Sodium can enhance the absorption of amino acid and storage of carbohydrates in our bodies. Because of the effects it can do to the cellular fluid, you are to expect that sodium can add to gain weight which lessens muscles to strain and injure soft tissues.

3. Train.

If you really wish to have muscle gain, you have to work on some exercises which need resistance like dumbbells that are considered as free weights. They would train your muscles in the ancillary portion to build a mass that will be compounded on them. Dumbbells can be versatile and at the same time useful for building muscles because of the range of motion you can exert when you carry them.

Gain Muscle and Eliminate Fat Tips on How to Do It

It is a fact that having those love handles and that beer belly as well as those man boobs can be quite embarrassing. If you want a body that you can be proud of and a body that you can show off whenever you are at the beach, then you may want to start working out.

So, what are the proper workout routines to burn fat and gain muscles?

Basically, the best muscle burning technique is through cardiovascular exercises. This helps in burning a lot of fat and calories which will significantly help in weight loss. Diet is also an important factor in order for you to lose fat and in most cases this is the most difficult part of weight loss.

Dieting doesn't mean that you have to starve yourself in order for you to lose fat. Eating right is.

What this means is that you need to eat less fatty foods and eat more foods that your body needs in order to function everyday. Eat foods that have plenty of fiber and in order to promote muscle growth, eat food with plenty of protein, such as beef.

You should also decrease the amount of carbohydrates you eat everyday. By reducing at least 25 percent of the total carbohydrates you eat everyday, you will see that it will give you a lot of difference when it comes to losing weight and burning off fat.

Doing a lot of cardiovascular exercises will also help in burning off fat. Every morning before breakfast, try to at least go jogging or walk for 30 minutes. This will significantly improve your weight as well as your body. By exercising before you eat breakfast, you will be able to turn on your metabolism rate and make it a lot faster. This means that you will be able to burn fat a lot more efficiently than not exercising in the morning at all.

Eating breakfast is also important as it helps jumpstart your metabolism rate. Always remember that it is advisable that you eat your breakfast. It actually helps in weight loss.

Also, when you reach the gym, it is still advisable to perform cardiovascular exercises. Try running for at least 15 minutes on the treadmill and it will burn at least a hundred to a hundred and fifty calories.

After doing cardiovascular exercises, it is now time to develop your muscles with weights. For maximum muscle gain, you might want to use as much free weights as you can. Try to minimize the use of the machine as the machines only focuses on the primary muscle and not the supporting muscles. If you want to gain muscle mass, it is recommended that you should strengthen the supporting muscles too. This will help in muscle growth. In fact, if you don't strengthen the supporting muscles, you will end up not being able to promote the primary muscles to grow.

These are some of the things that you have to remember about fat loss and muscle gain. Muscles burn fat and by exercising, you will be able to promote muscle growth and at the same time, promote fat loss. With these tips in mind and following it, you can be sure that you will be able to get rid of that fat and develop a body that you can be proud of.

Gain Muscles the Right Way The Facts about Body Building

As an ultra skinny person, you will find it very hard to gain muscles. If you think that spending a lot of time in the gym and doing long workouts will be able to help you gain muscles, you better think again. Although this may work, you have to consider that there are incorrect ways to do it and there are correct ways to do it.

By sticking to the principles of body building, you will be able to get the results you want in no time at all. So, if you are ever wondering why you can't gain muscles besides the fact that you spend a lot of time in the gym, here are some tips that will be able to enlighten you.

First of all, some people think that lifting weights rapidly will get them to gain muscles at a much efficient rate. However, what this does is exactly the opposite. You have to remember that in body building, you need to do each exercise in slow controlled movements. Fluidity is the key to exercising. This is because slow controlled movements encourage maximum muscle contractions, which means more efficient muscle building.

A few hours before and after you hit the gym, eat foods with high protein content. This will strengthen your muscles more and it encourages muscle tissue repair, which means that you will be able to gain muscles faster. Some people go on a diet and never eat anything before and after they go to the gym. This is a mistake. Besides, where will you be able to get the energy for all that heavy lifting?

Another mistake is exercising the same muscles everyday. This will do exactly the opposite when you want to gain muscle mass. Always remember that rest is the key to muscle gain. Always give the muscles you worked out today at least one or two days rest. For example, if you worked out the back and biceps today, never do the same exercises the next day. Give it time to repair itself and build more muscle tissues.

You need to remember that you don't gain muscles when you are working out. You injure it. When you rest, the body will compensate for the muscle tissue injury by producing more muscle tissues. The result is muscle gain. Resting is the best way to repair muscle tissues so get plenty of rest.

Every time you hit the gym, always go for heavier weights. However, don't try to lift weights that are too heavy for you that you can't complete a set and don't go for weights that are too light that it doesn't provide contractions in your muscles.

These are the things that you have to remember about body building. Always keep in mind that going to the gym everyday will not cut it. If you want to gain muscles, then you have to properly exercise each muscle group, eat the right kinds of food, and also get plenty of rest.

Remember these tips and you can be sure that you will be able to gain muscle in no time at all. Try exercising two muscle groups in one day and exercise two different muscle groups on the other day. Or, if you really want to be sure about your body building program, you might want to consult a professional trainer. They will be able to help you out with what kind of body building program and exercises that is right for you.

Gaining Muscle in your Gut, the Dream Six Pack Abs

More than having a spectacular looking chest muscles, a bulging biceps and triceps combo, most people would definitely want a well toned and sculpted six pack abs. The problem though is that the stomach muscles is one of the most difficult to develop. Well not really, they are developed as the same rate as the other muscles are, but, because body fat can also be very difficult to get rid off in that area, for stomach muscles to easily be seen, you first have to get rid of your body fat in that area.

There are so many body builders who get easily discouraged because after all their hard work they are not able to see any developments. Little do they know, their stomach muscles are already progressing, but they are not able to see the progress as there are fats covering the muscles in that area. Most of them would just get discouraged and abandon the idea. So what needs to be done then? First things first, one must not be easily discouraged, you may already have great looking abs underneath all your stomach fats, so the common thing to do is to get rid of the fats to make them show.

What you need to do to eliminate fat is to do some hard hitting cardio exercises to eliminate the fat and sweat them all away. To do this, you must go in a diet, no, I'm not saying starving yourself, all you need to do is to burn away all the calories you ingest. So even if you pig out, it's okay all you need to do is to burn them all away, that is if you're willing to do cardio exercises half of the day.

So to avoid this predicament, keep away from foods heaping with saturated fats. A diet of pizzas, burgers and processed meat will do you no wonders, that is if your goal is setting the record for the heaviest person on the whole world or the fastest weight gain in a year.

Some of the best cardio exercises you can do won't even cost you a cent. The point here is to get your heart rate running at full nitro mode. Running, swimming, biking and maybe just going up and down the stairs at a fast pace can easily help in achieving your goal. Anything that can make you sweat and get your heart rate pumping will do the job. Doing this for about 15 to 30 minutes each day will show significant results. In no time at all, you will be burning body fat in no time at all.

Cardio exercises though will only work if you already have developed abs. So if you don't, you should integrate exercises that will shock your stomach muscles to develop. Crunches in different forms would be ideal. Avoid doing the same exercises everyday as the muscles may get accustomed to them and just adapt to them inhibiting muscle growth. In one day concentrate on the center muscles, the next day work on the side muscles.

Also try to increase the intensity of your workout. Use weights if possible. This is so that the muscles don't easily get accustomed to the exercise and make it comfortable with the process.

Gaining Muscles Takes Time... How Long

Some people think that gaining muscles is as easy as popping a can of soda. Well it's not that easy. You have to wait for months to see acceptable results. You have to consider a lot of things if you're aiming for firm and perfect muscles. First, the things that you eat must be healthy in order for you to sustain your body's exertion in gaining mass. You have to observe the proper ways of exercise and your muscle growth should be assessed. Here, you will know whether or not you have the appropriate genes to be able to build and gain muscles more quickly than the other.

If you don't see anything that fits your type, worry not, because this is just one of those many factors that can determine the duration of muscle growth. It is also helpful that you know the type of body that you have and the kind of muscle that you wanted to build because through this knowledge, you will know the right kind of exercise and nutritional program that will suit your body's requirement to grow.

There are three body types and the specific characteristic underneath it.

Type 1 – Endomorph
As an endomorph, you have a naturally large frame for a body and a round face with wider hips and bigger bones but has slower metabolism. This is the type of body that gains body fat and weight easily but also the type of person can have the capability to gain mass in a quicker way. The only

problem that you will encounter is that your muscles tend to hide under the fat that you have which will make you look bulkier and clumsier. Even if you develop six packs, it wouldn't be that prominent because of your fat tummy.

That is why, you have to grow muscles and at the same time burn the unnecessary fats for your muscles to be revealed and more defined. End point: you have to spend more time inside the gym because aside from wanting to refined muscles, you have to burn those fats away.

Type 2 – Mesomorph

These are the persons who are naturally blessed with a body that has a wider shoulder and a more muscular body. You also have a small waist and a frame fit for entering athletic competitions. Because your body has lower contents of body fat, you also have an increase metabolic rate. Because of your general predisposition, you can pack those muscles and develop it really fast. You have the tendency to naturally excel in any kind of sport that you want because your body can easily adapt to it.

Type 3 – Ectomorph

Skinny type and small muscles that is what you are. You have a high level of metabolism with narrow hips, waist and shoulders. With this kind of stature, you will find it hard to gain on some muscles and weight. No matter how much effort you put in eating, you'll still get the skinny frame. This kind of frame will make it harder for you to build some mass because your proteins and fats don't last long.

People who fall under one of these criteria can have the specific unilateral characteristics or others may have mix of it. Either way, you now know that it will greatly depend on your body type and on how long you can gain muscles.

How to Double Your Muscle Gain

A body building workout program should be tailored to your body type in order to get positive results. You have to remember that your body is different from other people. You have different metabolism rate and you also have a different body structure that will require a different body building program. If your friend has a great body building program, don't expect that the same program will work for you.

One mistake that most people make when it comes to body building is that they stick to a program that doesn't work at all. Besides, if you see that your body building program is not working, why should you stick to it at all? Why should you keep on doing it? It's a complete waste of time and energy.

Try to give a work out program a week or two. This way, you will be able to see if there are any improvements or not. Do not use the same work out program for three months if you don't see any positive results right after two weeks of using the program.

Here are some tips that will be able to maximize efficiency when you work out and also maximize your body building exercises.

First of all, you need to remember that half reps will not cut it. Do only full reps even if it is strenuous. However, you have to avoid overtraining at the same time. Always remember that in body building, resting is very important. Try to rest for at least a day between workout sessions. This way, you will be able to give your muscles the rest it needs in order to grow.

You also need to keep in mind that when you go on a body building exercise, you are deliberately injuring your muscles. What you are actually doing is injuring your muscles in order for it to grow. When you injure your muscles through body building, you are letting the body adjust to your activities and let it grow stronger and bigger muscle tissues. This is what actually happens when you go body building.

If you are overweight or you are fat, then you have to remember that the best way to reduce fat is by adding cardiovascular exercises in your body building program. Cardiovascular exercises burn calories and fat as it is an aerobic exercise. Weight lifting is considered to be anaerobic exercises which mean that it burns sugar.

The correct execution of the exercises is also very important in promoting muscle growth. A lot of people make a mistake of doing each exercise too fast. Some just allows the weight to drop. This is a mistake. Going slow on each repetition is actually more beneficial as you are concentrating. For example, if you are doing standing barbell curls, don't do it too fast. Instead, lift the barbell up until you fully contract your biceps and slowly lower it down to the starting position. The lowering motion actually is more effective than the curling motion or the lifting motion in promoting muscle growth.

With slow, smooth, and controlled motion, you will concentrate on the muscles more which means that it is more effective in promoting muscle growth.

These are just some of the many ways on how you can gain muscle at a fast rate. Always remember that with the proper diet, proper execution of the exercises, and the right amount of rest, you will be able to get the results you want fast.

Increase Metabolism for Gaining Muscle

A well balanced diet and the proper workout regimen always work hand in hand in gaining muscle. If you are going for a well sculpted body with fine cuts and muscle definition, then you need to lose all the unwanted body fats in your body. This doesn't mean though that you have to starve yourself, on the contrary, you need to eat more, more of the types of food that can increase your metabolism.

Dieting is not just about eating small amount of food, it's more about having the proper eating habits. Remember the food pyramid? It's all about knowing what to eat more and what to eat less. Eat plenty of whole grains, vegetables, and fruits. Limit your intake of fatty and sugary foods. But in gaining muscle, you need to have the proper amount of calories which will help fuel muscle growth and development. So preparing a special diet is in order. Getting the services of a dietician or nutritionist can help you a lot.

At first you may think that you are not losing weight fast enough. But if your goal is gaining muscle, then losing weight is not as fast as it would be when working out for the purpose of losing weight alone. This is because in a lose weight and gain muscle program, your weight reduction in body fat will be appended by the weight gain of muscle growth. This is a good thing as your weight will not be based on how much body fat you have but by the muscles you have gained.

Increasing your metabolism is essential in your workout as this is the process that boosts and generates energy for the body to help in developing your muscles. As you develop a good diet, you will be able to tweak the maximum efficiency of your body in producing energy which is very much needed when you are working out. Even all your normal activities like walking, sleeping, breathing and plain sitting require energy, so imagine how much would be needed when working out strenuously?

For gaining muscle, you will indeed be working out strenuously. You will be doing lots of strength training and weight lifting. Heavy weights will greatly help you in developing muscles. This can get very tiring though, so you really have to be determined in keeping up with your program. A professional trainer will be able to provide you a specialized strength training that will be able to maximize your training time.

Your attitude towards developing yourself will also make a big impact. You must be persistent and patient. Muscles don't grow overnight. In fact, you won't really be able to notice them in the first few weeks. But don't be discouraged, just stick with your program. The body and muscle pains you feel after working out is a clear sign that what you're doing is working. Feel the burn.

So there it is, the basics in gaining muscle and losing weight. It's not just about breaking a sweat, its all about laser targeting all the aspects involved. A good diet (proper eating habits), and a rigid strength training and workout regimen, will definitely set you on the road to losing weight, gaining muscle, and basically bring out a better looking and healthier you.

Muscle Gain Benefits for Women

Women who are into fit slim and anorexic bodies won't even consider looking at the sides of healthy exercise. Again, muscle gain is not only meant for those who wanted to have muscles but also for those who wanted to maintain a healthy lifestyle. Living is not just eating right and achieving the right sleep hours. You have to make your body work in order to get firmer and increase your body's circulating status.

Nowadays, there are a lot of women who go into body building to achieve a body that is familiar among the masses. Besides, bodybuilding can contribute to a more positive energy. It gives out negative aspects of work and stressors and changes it with a rejuvenating feeling.

Really, there are no bad effects if you tighten up those muscles every once in a while. Generally, people wanted to exert muscle growth in order to gain, lose and increase. What are the different reasons why women wanted to get into bodybuilding?

Reason # 1 – Burn unnecessary fats
For women who weigh more than their expected size, bodybuilding is a way to decrease the fats inside their body. This will decrease their chances of getting diseases and disorders like liver problems and heart problems which is the end result of being fat or eating unhealthy. Some women who are successful in burning fats tend to produce muscles that are also

prevalent in men. And because men has an increased level of testosterone, it is expected that they would have the greater bulk of muscles compared to women. Women, on the other hand, are toned easier.

Reason # 2 – Competition purposes
For women who are into bodybuilding, one of the major reasons why they wanted to gain muscles is to join in bodybuilding competitions. By winning in competitions like these, women challenged and at the same time satisfied with themselves. For athletes, being skinny is not an option because it is only applicable to models that need to maintain flesh and bones just to stay in the business.

In order to understand your goals, you have to set them up. In case that you wanted to go into competitions, you have to lay down your plans that are suitable in achieving your goal. Your goal is to bulk up which means that you have to go into careful sculpturing of your body. Your diet must be at a limit and calories should be maximized in order to give your body additional energy for muscles to grow.

Bodybuilding has become popular to women because of the personal benefits that they expect to gain. Weight lifting has also become popular. In order to be fit in all aspects, one much first practice exercising parts so that it won't strain the body. Soon, you will notice how your body can adapt to the exercises and you can also add up to the minimal exercise.

When you have reached the desired body, all you have to do is maintain it.

It is also important that one introduces different exercises in order to let your body experience other exercises and let your body tone even more. With these benefits, there are more and more women getting hooked with muscle gain and some even promote the trend in order to continue muscle strengthening and growth.

Muscle Gain Free Weights vs. Machines

A lot of people debate about which one is effective when it comes to exercising and producing muscles. They often debate whether machines are more effective or free weights. Basically, barbells and free weights are classified as free weights. On the other hand exercises that have pulleys or cables to help you lift the weight are machines.

In order to gain muscles, you need to focus more on free weight exercises. For all machine enthusiasts out there, you might rethink about which one is more effective. Free weights are indeed more effective in promoting muscle growth. Although the exercises here are much more difficult to execute because nothing is actually assisting you to employ the correct execution, this fact alone is why free weight exercise is much more effective.

Free weight exercises are able to stimulate most of the muscle fibers as possible. This is impossible to do with a machine. Why?

Basically, machines lack in promoting stabilizers and synergist muscle development. Basically, these two muscles are what support the main muscles when you are performing a complex lift. For example, if you need to do bench presses, you need to be able to make use of the stabilizers and the synergist muscles in order for you to achieve lift. And, you need lots of it. If you bench press using a machine, it will not really need any assistance from the stabilizers as the machine itself is already supporting your main muscles.

Machines basically fail to stimulate the muscles around the area you are working on, which are the stabilizers. You need to remember that in order for your main muscles to grow, the stabilizers should be strong. And, the only way to do this is by doing as much free weight exercises as you can.

Free weight exercises, such as squats, dumbbell presses, dumbbell fly, bench presses, bent over dumbbell row, and others put a lot of stress in the supporting muscle groups, which is why you get tired really fast doing free weight exercises. However, even if you do get tired really fast, you will gain more muscles and you will become a lot stronger at a very fast rate.

You can include machine exercises in your program but you need to do it after you execute all the free weight exercises. This way, you will be able to take advantage of the strength you have on free weight exercises and not deplete it on machine exercises.

If you are a beginner, concentrate on lighter weights. Your primary goal is not muscle gain yet. You first need to properly execute the free weight exercises you have in your program in order for you to move on to heavier weights.

Concentrate on strengthening the supporting muscles first and when it is able to support the weight you are lifting and that you are able to execute the free weight exercises properly, then it's time for you to concentrate on the primary muscles.

Also, in order to build muscle mass, you need to lift heavier weights. What heavy means is that weights that are challenging for you and weights that you will be able to lift with 8 to 12 repetitions for 3 sets. If you can do more than 15 repetitions before temporary failure sets in, then it will be considered as light weight.

Remember these tips and you can be sure that you will be able to gain muscles fast. Always remember that one of the keys to muscle gain is to strengthen the supporting muscles. And, only doing free weight exercises will be able to do this efficiently.

Muscle Gain in a Jiffy

Apart from what others would say, there are only three important things that you have to know in order to gain muscle fast. But first, you have to have a lot of discipline sliding through your veins in order to start a program that will benefit your well-being. You should have proper nutrition and diet, an exercise or training program, and lots of rest. Easy, right? So, just pay attention and you'll be all set to enjoy muscles in a jiffy.

Know your nutritional status

Body building is more on adhering to the proper diet. Training those abs and muscles would only be secondary. No kidding. Proper promotion of nutrition and diet can greatly help and not put your dreams of gaining the mass that you need in jeopardy. Unless you set the proper eating habit, your program will never work.

If you're stuck with the conventional habit of eating, then change it. It is said that instead of eating meals in large amounts, you can do it by small frequent meals. You can eat 3 to 4 times a day but in small amounts.

Furthermore, you would want to keep head track on the things that you eat. You can do this for a week. Tracking will keep you update with what you are putting inside your system. You will soon figure out the calories, proteins, fats, etc. Eventually, you will know what to increase or decrease in your diet. After you have figured out what your diet should be, you have to enroll in a rigid training program that offers less time for more muscles.

Enroll in a muscle fitness program

A muscle fitness program will be helpful for you to increase the chances of getting those muscles more efficiently and effectively. Don't settle with the things that you would want to do inside the gym because that would be insufficient. There are several programs that enable you to gain or loose weight.

Once you have chosen the muscle fitness program, you have to discipline yourself on being consistent. You should follow the schedule that was given to you by your gym instructor. The usual work out schedule would only consist of 3 or 4 days every week. Not unless you are enrolled in an advanced program, you have no reason why you can't do the exercise daily.

Always stick to the plan. Never let a day pass without working out. One more thing, you have to avoid exercises which will isolate you. You have to stick to the tried and tested, basic compounds of exercises and movements.

Rest

After a tiring day at the gym, it's time to give your muscles some rest. They need it bad. Fact is, muscle growth happens after gym which is during rest periods. When you weight lifts, you muscles tend to extend and fibers are torn apart. The process of repair is the reason why your muscles become stronger and bigger.

You can rest your muscles by simply sleeping. You should have at least 6 to 7 hours of sleep. This will do you more than extending hours inside the gym. After sleep, you'll realize that you are more energized and alert and you'll find your self satisfied with the results.

Do not stick to the thoughts that muscle gain is one heck of a hassle because it's not. You should not result to complicating things in terms of gaining muscles. You should have all three in order to speed up the formation of your dream muscles.

Steroids used for Muscle Gain can be Dangerous

Steroids are somewhat considered as synthetic derivatives found in male sex hormones which are known to man as testosterone and are usually taken in order to improve the size and strength of muscles. Though some may not admit it but there are a lot of bodybuilders and also known personalities that uses steroids in order to get muscle gain. Testosterones are the ones that are responsible for building muscles and tissues focused for the males. Steroids are the ones that boost the building process of muscles by enhancing the number of testosterone in the body.

Steroids also affect the growth of organs for reproductive in order to enlarge the penile length and prevent the development of facial and pubic hair. Some people would opt to using steroids because of the rate or degree of faster mass increase and fat loss. Despite that, steroids are also believed to cause several effects which contribute problems to the body which is usually the reason why it is incorporated in bodybuilding phases. Psychological and physical damage can be the effects of steroids in the body and this reason overshadows the need for superficial disadvantages.

Steroids are also used in healthcare facilities to reduce the effects of any inflammatory process going inside the body. It can also cause some symptoms of certain diseases to be diminished. Inhalers made from steroids decreases deaths due to asthma and other respiratory obstruction; injections of steroids can be useful in treating pains from ligaments and joints. However, steroids are also responsible for making the body's immune system less active which is why it is considered as an anti-inflammatory drug.

Effects of abused steroid use can result to the following side effects:

• Increased blood pressure

• Reduce the level of high density lipoprotein which is considered as good fats

• Obliteration of the liver

• Testicle contraction in males

• Uterus and breast contraction in females

• Impotency and infertility in both females and males

• Mood swings that are irrepressible which includes belligerence and irritability

No matter how you see it, steroid use should be avoided because of the possible adverse effects that it might contribute to your body in the long run. The effect is irreparable. It is more advisable that you be included in an exercise program that is steadily healthy, educated, and gives the chance for the person to improve muscle growth in the most natural way.

After mentioning these side effects, do you still want to do it the hard way or the easy way out which can be pretty life threatening. Some of the other side effects due to muscle gaining that can be acquired through the use of steroids are:

• Anaphylactic shock
• Unusual bleeding or hemorrhage
• Unpleasant odor of breath
• Persistent headaches
• Cholesterol levels which are fluctuating
• Fetal damage (if pregnant)
• Regurgitation with blood
• Diarrhea
• Morbid fluid accumulation or edema
• Excessive calcium levels or low calcium levels
• Injuries that are delayed
• Impotence
• Irregularity in menstrual periods
• Jaundice
• Breast swelling or soreness that may eventually lead to breast cancer
• Atrophy of the testicles
• Injuries of the ligaments
• Stones in gallbladder
• Nausea and vomiting

- Blood poisoning or septic shock
- Abnormal urinary retention or excretion
- Painful reproductive organs (male)
- Insomnia
- Problems regarding sexuality

Techniques for Building Muscles and Getting Results

It is a fact that body builders gain muscles at a very fast rate. So, just how do they do this and why can't you have the same results? Basically, body builders know the techniques on how to gain muscles at a very fast rate. In fact, two months before a body building competition, you will see that they have body fat and their muscles aren't really defined. However, when the day for the competition comes, you will see that they are incredibly ripped.

So, just what are the secrets for gaining muscles at a very fast rate?

Actually, it's not really a secret. You may not be properly doing the exercises and following your program by the book. A lot of people make mistakes when it comes to building muscles and gaining muscle mass.

For example, a lot of people think that doing each exercises at a very fast rate will increase their muscle mass. However, this is a sure fire way to slow down muscle growth. Slow rep speed is one of the keys to muscle growth. Slow is good when it comes to lifting weights. For example, when you do bench presses, make sure that you lift the barbell in a slow, controlled, and smooth movement. The slower you go, the more muscle contractions there is. And, with more muscle contractions, the more you promote muscle strain which will in turn promote muscle growth.

Another key to muscle growth is control. Never throw your weight around and never ever throw the weights you are lifting around too. This is not only inefficient when it comes to promoting muscle growth, but it is also dangerous and may result in muscle and joint injuries.

Lots of people think that eating lots of meat is bad. However, it is only bad if you are a couch potato. With exercise, meat, especially beef, will actually do you good than harm especially when it comes to muscle growth. Meat contains protein and protein promotes muscle growth and muscle tissue repair.

Resting is another key to muscle growth. A lot of people think that exercising the same muscles everyday will promote muscle growth. However, this is exactly the complete opposite of what you are aiming for. Instead of promoting muscle growth, it will make the muscle smaller. You have to remember that whenever you work out, you injure your muscles.

Injuring the muscles means that the body will repair the muscles by replacing it with larger and much stronger muscle tissues. And, the best way to promote muscle tissue repair and muscle growth is by resting. It usually takes two to three days for the muscles to regenerate. So, never exercise the same muscles everyday. Give it a rest for at least two days.

These are some of the secret techniques employed by body builders all over the world and these are the techniques on how they gain muscles rapidly. So, if you also want to gain muscles, you might want to keep these tips in mind.

Always remember that proper execution, control, high protein diet, and rest are some of the ways on how to promote muscle growth fast. With these tips in mind, you can be sure that you will gain muscle and strength in no time at all.

A lot of people don't know for a fact that there is a right way to gain muscles and there are wrong ways to do it. And, many people do the wrong way and ends up getting frustrated as they can't get the results they want.

Doing it the wrong way will not only mean slow results, but it will also mean injuries that may hinder you from exercising regularly and correctly.

Body building is also considered as science. There are correct procedures for it in order for you to get the results you want.

First of all, a lot of people think that in order to gain muscle, they need to exercise the same muscles everyday. This is in fact a mistake. It will do the exact opposite of what you want. Instead of gaining muscles, you will in fact lose muscles.

Lifting weights does not make your muscles bigger. It injures it. So, when you lift weights, you are deliberately injuring your muscles. So, which part of the exercises makes the muscles bigger? Well, you'll be surprised to know that resting is what makes the muscles bigger.

For example, if you worked out your biceps, you are deliberately injuring it. When it is injured, the body will react by producing more muscle tissues in the injured part in this case, the biceps. The fastest way to repair muscle and gain muscle tissues is if you sleep. This is the time where muscle repair is the most efficient.

So, the key to muscle gain is to actually get enough rest after working out. It is not advisable to work out the same muscle group everyday as it will not efficiently gain muscle as it takes at least two days of good sleep to fully replace the injured muscles with much bigger and stronger muscle tissues. So, when you work out, try providing some intervals on what muscle group you have to work out on each day.

A good example would be working out the chest and triceps on day one, back and biceps on day two, and legs and shoulders on day three. The abdominal muscles should be worked out everyday.

Try to provide four to five exercises on each of the muscle groups with 3 sets with 10 repetitions each.

However, you might want to change the exercises for each muscle group every two weeks in order to avoid the plateau where the muscles will get so used to the exercises that it will not grow any larger.

Another mistake that people do when it comes to body building is that they often execute the exercises at a very fast rate. They may think that this is a more efficient way to build muscles, but it's actually not. You have to execute the exercises in a smooth, controlled, and slow motions in order to promote maximum muscle contractions.

These are just some of the correct ways to gain muscle. Always remember that muscle gain is not just about lifting weights but there is a system that you need to follow in order for you to gain muscles efficiently and get the results you want at the soonest time possible. In fact, it is very possible to gain muscles in just a matter of weeks. Do it right and you will see fast results.

The Right Workout Routine for Gaining Muscles

Have you ever been to the gym lately and you feel like a skinny geek among those guys who had huge muscles? If you do, then don't let those guys intimidate you. You have to remember that they have been through on what you are going through. They were also skinny or fat once and they worked hard to get the body they have today. In fact, they may even help you get the results you want if you ask them politely.

They may give you some tips on how to gain muscles fast and some of these tips may actually work. However, if you really want to gain muscles fast, then here are some of the right workout routines that you should follow in order for you to get that serious muscle that you have always wanted to have.

First of all, you need to remember that in order to gain muscles you should emphasize more on free weight exercises. Machine exercises may seem to be appealing as it lowers the risk of injury. However, you have to consider that in order to gain muscles, you need to strengthen the supporting muscles first, such as the synergist and the stabilizers. Machines don't do this as the machines themselves act as a stabilizer.

Free weights will require your muscles as well as the supporting muscles to work really hard. This is why you will get tired a lot quicker when doing free weight exercises.

If you hear someone say that you need to exercise the same muscle group everyday, then don't take this advice. This will slow down the growth rate of your muscles. You have to remember that working out means that you are actually injuring or tearing your muscles. If you do this everyday, it will lead to the deterioration of your muscles.

So, why work out if you are only tearing or injuring your muscles? You have to remember that when you injure your muscles, the body will react by replacing or adding more muscle tissues to strengthen the injured muscles. This means muscle growth or an increase in the muscle mass. And, the best time for your muscles to grow is by resting or sleeping.

Try exercising different parts of the body each day. For example, on day one, you might want to exercise your chest and triceps. On day two, exercise the back and biceps. And, on day three, exercise the legs and shoulders. On each day, always exercise your abdominal muscles with sit ups, crunches and other abdominal exercises.

After day three, you should rest the next day and after that, start again with day one. Do this for two weeks and change the exercises to avoid reaching the plateau where your muscles become so used to the exercises that it will not grow anymore.

On each muscle group, try to create 4 to 5 exercises. For example, for the chest, do bench presses, inclined dumbbell presses, lying dumbbell fly, and cable crossovers. For each exercise do 10 reps and 3 sets each.

These are the things that you need to remember about muscle gain and the correct exercise routines for it. Always remember that proper execution is the key to muscle growth. Resting is also very important as well as diet.

The Three Essentials in Gaining Muscle Big Time

Tired of looking in the mirror and not seeing the superman that you want to be? Do you crave to have the Hollywood hunk abs and biceps? Most of us do, but the entire process of getting muscles is simply strenuous. Hollywood actors have all the time in the world to bulk up and have an army of trainers and experts to help them, and this could cost an arm and a leg. But even with those aspects gaining muscle is not going to happen if there is no determination.

For one thing, it's undeniably extremely hard to gain muscles; there is no doubt about it. You have to invest a lot of time and patience. You must have full commitment to meet your goal. But aside from just going under a rigorous training program, there are certainly numerous aspects one must consider. All of these aspects together can help make a program effective and let you achieve your goal at the fastest time possible.

Here are the three essential steps in those aspects which can greatly determine the success a person will have in gaining muscles.

A) Have the proper diet - A lot of people misconstrue the word "diet." A lot of them think that diet equates to starving one's self. A diet means that a person, depending on his goal, has the proper and correct food intake. If you are thinking of gaining muscle and weight, then eating more calories than what you would be expecting to burn when you have an extensive workout would be necessary to fuel the growth of muscles. You will need to have a balanced intake of protein, soy and fats. A nutritionist or dietician will be able to help you know what is good for you.

B) Develop a strength training program – Muscles are built when they are regularly pushed to the limit. Perpetual couch potatoes don't build muscles, they grow guts. You must develop a strength training program which would make you lift weights that you won't be able to easily lift. This should go on until you progress to heavier weights. Your muscle will react to the heavy lifting and will grow to compensate for the needed strength to lift the heavy weights. As you move on to heavier weights, the muscle will continually grow for strength compensation.

C) Have sufficient rest – Contrary to popular belief, your muscles don't grow while your lifting weights, they grow when they are resting. As you work out, your muscles are strained and flexed to their limit, especially if you lift the proper weights. When you go to sleep, the damage done to the muscles will be repaired and this is when they grow. 8 hours of sleep daily is the minimum requirement for proper muscle growth.

Some people add supplements and medications which can also help in growth promotion of muscles. There are now many of them available in the market, make sure though that they are legal and safe for you.

So there it is the three basic essentials one would need to follow in gaining muscle. Commit to these basics and you will see that all your efforts will not go to waste. Now get off that couch and start pumping iron.

Things You Need To Know To Effectively Gain Muscle

Have you ever wanted to have that great looking body that you can be proud of? Do you want to have big muscles or just a greatly defined body that everyone will admire? Well, you have to remember that just lifting weights in the gym is not enough for you to gain muscles.

You have to remember that there is different exercise programs suited for different people. There are specific exercises for losing weight and burning fat, and there are also exercises designed for weight gain. You will even see exercises for strength training.

If you want to gain muscle mass, then you have to do body building exercises. In body building exercises, you will have a series of exercises in a day and a different one the next day. Usually, body building exercises will have 3 exercise days. On each day, different muscle groups will be targeted. However, the abs should be exercised everyday as this is considered to be one of the most important muscle groups that you need to exercise and it is also one of the hardest.

On day one, the chest and triceps are the muscle groups that you need to exercise. For the chest exercise, you will need to do at least four to five different chest exercises that will target different parts of the chest. The same goes for the triceps. Do 10 repetitions of each exercise with 3 sets.

On day two, exercise the back and the biceps. Four exercises for the back and four for the biceps. Also, do 10 repetitions for each of the exercises for 3 sets.

On day three, exercise the leg, thigh, and butt muscles and the shoulders. Four exercise for the legs, and four for the shoulders. Also, for each exercise, do 10 repetitions with 3 sets.

On each day, you need to have four or five exercises for the abdominal muscles. Sit ups, and crunches are two of the exercises that you may want to

You have to remember that the key in gaining muscle mass is getting adequate rest and eating foods that are high in protein. When you exercise, you have to remember that you are injuring your muscles in a controlled way. When you injure your muscles, it will repair those injuries by adding more muscle tissues. And, in order for the muscles to repair itself, you need to let it rest. Eating foods that are rich in protein, such as beef and soya milk protein will be able to make the muscle repair process faster and also make it stronger.

This is why body building exercises have intervals when it comes to exercising each muscle group. It allows each of the muscle group to have enough time to repair itself.

It is also very important to remember that you should exercise every muscle group stated. Besides, you can't expect to have a great looking biceps, triceps or chest if the back can't support it. You also need to exercise your back in order for you to develop the chest, biceps, and triceps. Also, you have to exercise the shoulders in order for you to develop your arms. Everything is connected.

These are the things that you have to remember about body building or muscle gain. Always remember that resting is very important. Allow the muscles you exercised today to rest for two days. Get enough sleep and eat foods with high protein content and you will be able to gain muscle in no time at all.